The Lord Your Healer

Discover Him and Find His Healing Touch

Paul J. Bucknell

Books by Paul J. Bucknell

Allowing the Bible to speak to our lives today!

Overcoming Anxiety: Finding Peace, Discovering God

Life in the Spirit! Experiencing the Fullness of Christ

Reaching Beyond Mediocrity: Being an Overcomer

The Life Core: Discovering the Heart of Great Training

The Godly Man: When God Touches a Man's Life

Redemption Through the Scriptures

Godly Beginnings for the Family

Principles and Practices of Biblical Parenting

Building a Great Marriage

Christian Premarital Counseling Manual for Counselors

Relational Discipleship: Cross Training

Running the Race: Overcoming Sexual Lusts

The Bible Teaching Commentary on Genesis

The Bible Teaching Commentary on Romans

Life Transformation: A Monthly Devotional on Romans 12:9-21

Book of Romans: Bible Studies

Book of Ephesians: Bible Studies

Abiding in Christ: Walking with Jesus

Inductive Bible Studies in Titus

1 Peter Bible Study Questions: Living in a Fallen World.

Take Your Next Step into Ministry

The Lord Your Healer: Discover Him and Find His Healing

Training Leaders for Ministry

Satan's Four Stations: The Destroyer is Destroyed

Study Questions for Jonah: Understanding the Heart of God

Our Digital Libraries include these books as well as slides, handouts, audio/videos, and much more at: www.foundationsforfreedom.net

The Lord Your Healer

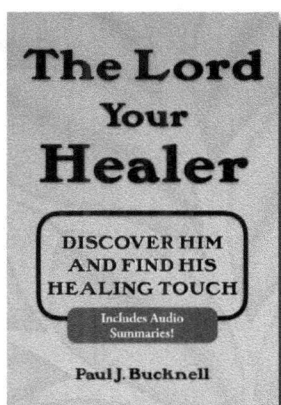

Paul J. Bucknell

Discover Him and Find His Healing Touch

The Lord Your Healer: Discover Him and Find His Healing Touch

Printed paperback:
ISBN-10: 1-61993-073-0
ISBN-13: 978-1-61993-073-5

Also as digital eBook
ISBN-10: 1-61993-074-9
ISBN-13: 978-1-61993-074-2

www.foundationsforfreedom.net
info@foundationsforfreedom.net

Pittsburgh, PA 15212 USA

The NASB Bible is used unless otherwise noted. Scripture quotations are taken from the New American Standard Bible®, Copyright © 1960, 1962, 1963, 1968, 1971, 1972, 1973, 1975, 1977, 1995 by The Lockman Foundation. Used by permission. (www.Lockman.org)

A Tribute

We give full praise to the Healer, the all-merciful Creator, who bestows an inordinate amount of mercy on us by extending life to those who languish under the heavy curse of disease and death, and in good time, sending His only Son, Jesus Christ, to suffer our disease and death so that we could have life eternal!

Thanks

I deeply appreciate the Lord for breaking into my stereotype answers on healing with His Word from Exodus 15:26 and illuminating my heart and mind. I am extremely grateful for my third daughter, Allison Bucknell, who so skillfully got this book off to the printers!

Table of Contents

An Introduction

My study on Exodus 15:26 has led me through completely unexpected learning experiences of healing. One of the key words in scripture, "life", all of a sudden took on a clarified meaning and promise. Healing was no longer simply a penchant cry from His people, but a pathway to know Him, the Healer, and even more, to gain eternal life through Jesus Christ.

While examining the material I had prepared, I was surprised to find answers to many key questions about healing, God, and the scriptures in the Exodus 15:26 text. I redesigned that study to be a book of questions and answers on healing so that we can be better equipped to powerfully communicate those answers. Each chapter also has a brief audio lesson, an extension of the reading you will find in this book, which I trust will cause you to dig deeper and to become more excited in the Lord, our Savior and Healer.

Although today's world regularly spites God's mercy, His Healing name, Jehovah Rophe, is beautiful. This book will hopefully serve as a resource to strengthen believers to see how powerful God's love is and that in no situation—even in great sickness and pain—do we ever need to be apologetic for God's actions, but satisfied and delighted.

May you be as blessed as I was in the discovery of these truths. And if you have any other questions on healing, please pass them my way!

Paul J. Bucknell

Pittsburgh, PA USA

July 2016

Jehovah Rophe

Jehovah Rophe, I am the Lord Your Healer (Ex 15:26)

And He said, 'If you will give earnest heed to the voice of the LORD your God, and do what is right in His sight, and give ear to His commandments, and keep all His statutes, I will put none of the diseases on you which I have put on the Egyptians; for I, the LORD, am your healer.' (Exodus 15:26)

Many of the unanswered questions regarding healing exacerbate the doubt that the secularists have regarding God's love and mercy. This study on Exodus 15:26 boldly reveals and explains God's statement, "I Myself am Your Healer," which is important when we consider the seeming rise in disease around us. "Why does He allow His children to suffer?" is just one of the questions we pose. Each of the tough questions we address in this book will be informed by a clear and powerful answer from this text. By studying each question and answer, you will gain a thorough biblical perspective on healing, and more importantly, you will find yourself drawn nearer the Healer.

The Lord Your Healer

Question #1

How can you be so sure that God is concerned about our lives if He allows so many health problems?

And He said, "If you will give earnest heed to the voice of the LORD your God, and do what is right in His sight, and give ear to His commandments, and keep all His statutes, I will put none of the diseases on you which I have put on the Egyptians; for I, the LORD, am your healer" (Ex 15:26).

A lot of the doubt surrounding God's concern for people exists because of the pain, suffering, and death we see everywhere we look. How can a loving God allow sickness and incurable diseases? So let us answer this question about health to combat the general mistrust people today have toward God. In Exodus 15:26, the Lord introduces Himself as the Healer, but I think if we take a look at this claim with a broader scope, we will see how it is revealing about God's love.

Exodus 15 starts with a few scenes from after God's deliverance of the Israelites from slavery in Egypt, the most powerful nation at that time. We see Miriam leading the sisters in praise for the amazing exodus. This natural outburst celebrates God's wonderful power, concern, and mercy. "And Miriam answered them, 'Sing to the LORD, for He is highly exalted; The horse and his rider He has hurled into the sea'" (Ex 15:21).

But the very next verses reveal a heart of complaint in the same people (Ex 15:22-25):

> 22 Then Moses led Israel from the Red Sea, and they went out into the wilderness of Shur; and they went three days in the wilderness and found no water. 23 And when they came to Marah, they could not drink the waters of Marah, for they were bitter; therefore it was named Marah.   24 So the people grumbled at Moses, saying, "What shall we drink?" 25 Then he cried out to the LORD, and the LORD showed him a tree; and he threw it into the waters, and the waters became sweet. There He made for them a statute and regulation, and there He tested them.

What is it that God did? He healed the waters and provided water to drink. What else did God do? He issued an awesome promise that provided a way for His people to avoid all the diseases of Egypt. The timing of the release of this promise is significant.

Think of a parent's relationship with their child. In what situation would they be inclined to reward their children with a promise of something nice like an ice-cream? Definitely not after their child has been complaining all day!

Parents love to think of nice things to do when their children are being sweet.

In what state do we find God's people here? They were acting like a bunch of ungrateful complainers. At this point, the Lord did not judge them, nor did He wait for them first to become sweet and humble; instead He offered them a beautiful word of radical promise. He told them the secret by which they could avoid the nasty diseases of Egypt.

> And He said, "If you will give earnest heed to the voice of the LORD your God, and do what is right in His sight, and give ear to His commandments, and keep all His statutes, I will put none of the diseases on you which I have put on the Egyptians; for I, the LORD, am your healer." (Ex 15:26)

What is God showing us about Himself in these interactions? We can see how quickly His children forget about the great things the Lord just did for them; they are already complaining about the way He leads them. Yet despite all of this, God offers them a sweet promise. The time and character of this promise reflect the wonderful love of God.

There are people, perhaps including you, who wonder if God cares. The depth of His care is made evident in this promise. God means the best for us. Always. "God so loved the world" (John 3:16). Though there are scoffers on our left and right, we should never doubt His care.

Now, we might not always understand why God does things the way He does them (like the testing in verse 25), but these moments stand out like bright, shining stars.

The same monumental grace can be found after Jesus' time. God never changes. "But God demonstrates His own love toward us, in that while we were yet sinners, Christ died for us." (Rom 5:6-8). While we were ungrateful, doubting sinners, God demonstrated His love to us. In other words, God loved us at our worst. He loved the Israelites at their worst, and He loves us at our worst. Nothing about God has changed.

Instead of doubting His love, we should instead be wondering why God has taken such serious steps to express His love for us. We might not understand all the technicalities of why Jesus suffered for us, but is it not a display of His care for us to send His Son Jesus to suffer for us? Before you make a quick conclusion that because God allows suffering and disease He doesn't love you, don't you think you should look behind His kind promise and acts of love? There is something going on behind the scenes that fully explains influenza, disease, and suffering that spreads across the face of the earth. Let's pause and thank Him for His love and invite Him to teach us more.

"But God demonstrates His own love
toward us, in that while we were yet
sinners, Christ died for us."
(Romans 5:8).

#1 Study Questions

How can you be so sure that God is concerned about our lives if He allows so many health problems?

1. Why do people sometimes question whether God really loves us?

2. When do you doubt God's love?

3. Why did the Israelites doubt God's love after crossing the Red Sea (Ex 15:22-25)?

4. Should they have questioned God's love? Why?

5. Why does the Lord 'test' His people at times (Ex 15:25)?

6. While considering the context, discuss how the Lord proves His love in Exodus 15:26.

7. After listing your doubts in God's love, repent from them, and find full forgiveness in Jesus.

8. Read Romans 5:6-8 and share how God showed His love through Jesus.

9. Can you identify with that love of God? If so, thank the Lord.

10. What piece of advice can you briefly state so that it will remind you not to doubt His love again?

The Lord Your Healer

Question #2

Why doesn't God just heal everybody, or at least all the Christians?

And He said, "If you will give earnest heed to the voice of the LORD your God, and do what is right in His sight, and give ear to His commandments, and keep all His statutes, I will put none of the diseases on you which I have put on the Egyptians; for I, the LORD, am your healer" (Ex 15:26).

This question might be a question of curiosity rather than of doubt. At times I ask myself, "Why did God do it this way?" or "Wouldn't it be better if He did it this way?"

For example, wouldn't it be magnificent if, when a person became a genuine believer in Christ, he or she would become instantly healed of their diseases? This would be proof that the gospel is true! But while God does heal, He doesn't always heal in one general way.

God works to provide a nice place for us. We can see that in His provision of the Garden of Eden. It was a fabulous place. He promises many wonderful comforts of life right after giving us the Ten Commandments in Deuteronomy 6-8. There is no doubt that God understands what we need to feel well and wants us to feel healthy and satisfied. There are other issues at hand, however.

If the Lord healed everyone, even after mankind had gone astray at the fall in the Garden of Eden, people would be well, but they would only be well until they perish and are left forever with the devil in the Lake of Fire (Rev 20:14-15). The judgment of death would still hang over our heads, but we wouldn't know it—until it was too late.

Sickness and disease are signs to alert us to our true situation; all is not well. When we are well, we do not usually consider our need for God or a Savior. Jesus Himself said that it is the sick who search for a doctor, not the healthy (Mark 2:17; Matt 9:12). The problem with modernity is the extent of comfort that it adds to our lives. People are so comfortable that they fall into a routine of self-care, which eliminates any thought of a need for a Savior; some even deny the existence of a supernatural being. Now, of course, when we are diagnosed with cancer, we are confronted with the fact that we are absolutely not in control, and so might remember the God of our childhood and seek His help. Calling out to God for healing is not a weakness but a healthy admittance to our true state of frailty.

If we all remained healthy until death, we would still meet up with God, but meet Him only as God the Judge. There is no mercy at the execution block.

Think of the Israelites here. After 400 years of exile in Egypt, they were rescued through miraculous means, but they willingly forgot all that after a few days of inconvenience in the desert after they crossed the Red Sea. If we, from day one, were fine, we wouldn't have a clue to the judgment coming upon us.

Disease and illness, as difficult as they are, are special messages from God to wake us up to our perilous condition—that we are indeed perishing and need a Savior. When you face years of chronic illness, your heart will be filled with more humility and the evil one will have limited success in using his deceit against you.

As much as we think the world would be better without sickness, it would not be. It would be a paradise for Satan, a world ripe with his lies laughing us all to hell. Instead of taking the easy way out and letting us think all is well, God sent His only Son, Jesus Christ, to live and suffer in this world, taking upon Himself our diseases so that we could be set free.

> Surely our sickness He Himself bore, And our sorrows He carried; Yet we ourselves esteemed Him stricken, smitten of God, and afflicted (Isaiah 53:4).

So instead of hiding our true condition from us, our gracious Father revealed how bad it was by the extreme judgment that Jesus bore. It is a startling view of our tragic situation, but because of His mercy, we can believe upon the Son of God, the Lamb who takes away the sin of the world, even while living under the curse of judgment, and seek a Savior where we can find true healing from the One who loves us dearly.

> "Behold, the Lamb of God who takes away
> the sin of the world!" (John 1:29)

#2 Study Questions

Why doesn't God heal everybody or at least all Christians?

1. When is the last time you heard someone say or infer that God does not exist because of the number of sick/ hurting or dead people? Describe what they said.

2. How do you take it when you hear people say that God is not a loving God?

3. If God provided full health for all of us, how would that really be hindering us?

4. Do you think it's possible that the pain and disease associated with sin sometimes prevent people from doing worse? Give an illustration.

5. How are sickness and disease messengers from God? What is the message?

6. Do you believe a good life on earth is more important than having eternal life? Explain.

7. Read John 1:29. How do we know that God didn't just make an unmerciful decision to allow disease and sickness?

8. How might you briefly answer a person who infers that God doesn't have mercy and love because He allows sickness?

The Lord Your Healer

Question #3

Why does it appear that God is the one who brings diseases upon the people?

And He said, "If you will give earnest heed to the voice of the LORD your God, and do what is right in His sight, and give ear to His commandments, and keep all His statutes, I will put none of the diseases on you which I have put on the Egyptians; for I, the LORD, am your healer" (Ex 15:26).

A question that troubles many people, including many believers, is God's association with disease. I remember one Christian speaking rather adamantly, "God never would bring sickness upon someone." People–even unbelievers–think they fully comprehend the love of God, but in fact, one cannot understand the love and mercy of God, until one understands the depth of our unworthiness to live even one more day.

There is more to this, though. Even in the Exodus 15:26 verse above, we see an association between God and the diseases of the world ("which I have put on the Egyptians"). The fact is, the Lord does oversee disease and final judgment. He is our Judge. God commanded man in the Garden of

Eden not to touch the forbidden fruit. The penalty of that disobedience was made clear before they went near this tree, but despite the warning and sure judgment, the man and woman ate the forbidden fruit and were judged, "for in the day that you eat from it you will surely die" (Gen 2:16-17).

The curse of judgment came on them because of their disobedience. We know that sin and judgment came because of man's disobedience, but the surprise is found in that Adam and Eve did not die immediately. God could have started anew, but He chose not to. This is a clue to the depth of God's mercy. The curse of death fell upon man; his life was as good as snuffed out, but it was at the same time extended. This is what we call healing.

Healing itself is the expression of God's mercy. God holds back death's invasion by renewing our bodies. And so, God's healing efforts become evident in the extension of life while we live under the curse. God doesn't need to perform any healing for mankind in order to be considered loving or kind. God is not at all obliged to bring mercy to us, because of our disobedience. We are the created. We are the debtors. We owe God our lives because we have exchanged it for disobedience.

That being said, God in His great mercy has extended His mercy to us by creating this tunnel of healing that protects us from the fury of death enveloping us. Healing is a measure of grace that extends our life. But what is the purpose of this extension of life?

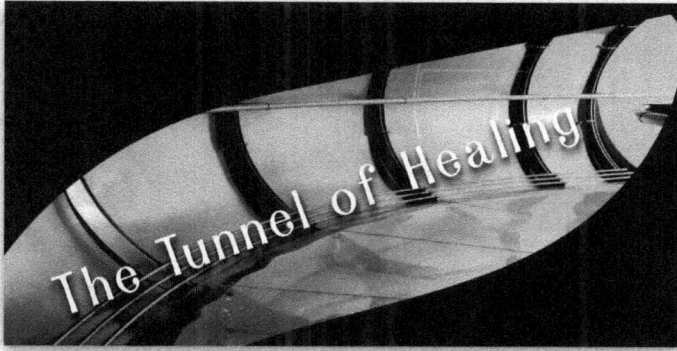

The Tunnel of Healing

God reached out to mankind and extended life and time itself so that He could send His only Son Jesus Christ to enter time, die for His people, and offer them eternal life. Life as we know it is really only an extension of the curse in a place where the full sentence of death is not executed. It creates a valuable but dwindling time period ("night is coming" John 9:4) in which we can pursue salvation; yet because this time is limited, we ought to live with a sense of urgency.

Healing, then, is a measure of God's grace extended to all so that His more perfect gift of salvation could be made on the cross and offered to mankind to believe and find eternal life. The pursuit of a better life on earth is not wrong but can create confusion over the purpose of the time that we have.

We are not called to live a comfortable life; we are called to live in such a way that people see God in our lives and are saved before the tidal wave of death and judgment come crashing down on all of us.

> "Truly, truly, I say to you, he who hears My
> word, and believes Him who sent Me, has
> eternal life, and does not come into
> judgment, but has passed out of death into
> life" (John 5:24).

#3 Study Questions

Why does it appear that God is the one who brings diseases upon the people?

1. Read Exodus 15:26 carefully. Do you think this verse suggests that God brings disease? Explain.

2. Some people cannot believe that God would bring sickness and disease on people. Are you one of them?

3. Why is God obligated to bring judgment on mankind?

4. Did the Lord warn Adam of the penalty of disobeying Him? What was it?

5. Could God have rightly and immediately destroyed them for disobedience? What about us?

6. Why did the Lord preserve their life and thus create mercy and a measure of health?

7. Some people see God's wrath and mercy as opposing each other but describe how our health is an example of their coexistence. Use the 'Tunnel of Healing' to explain.

8. How does Jesus' death demonstrate both God's wrath and mercy?

9. Read John 5:24. What does Jesus keep us from? What good does He bring?

10. Briefly, use the illustration 'Tunnel of healing' to explain God's love to someone who doubts because of sickness or suffering.

The Lord Your Healer

Question #4

What cure does God give that will keep us from diseases (Ex 15:26)?

And He said, "If you will give earnest heed to the voice of the LORD your God, and do what is right in His sight, and give ear to His commandments, and keep all His statutes, I will put none of the diseases on you which I have put on the Egyptians; for I, the LORD, am your healer" (Ex 15:26).

The Lord our Healer, gives us a glimpse into what it is that brings healing in Exodus 15:26: a list that provides the key to good health.

1. "Give earnest heed to the voice of the LORD your God"

2. "Do what is right in His sight"

3. "Give ear to His commandments"

4. "Keep all His statutes"

If the Israelites did these four things, the Lord who delivered them from the Egyptians, would be true to His Word and keep them from the diseases the Egyptians suffered. If we look carefully at these four lines, the four can be reduced to two instructions. In true Hebraic fashion, this repetition emphasizes the spoken message. Lines 1 and 3 both call the people to hear, that is, to actually gain the information they need to know. God is speaking. Is anyone listening? Lines 2 and 4 call them to follow through with what they heard. In Matthew, Jesus closed the Sermon on the Mount the same way: heed and do. Many people know the right thing to do, but do not do it. There may be many reasons they don't follow through, but the fact remains: disobedience is disobedience.

Many people disobey because they doubt God's will is good. They still long for the world, just like the Israelites who escaped Egypt longed to return to their oppression. "We remember the fish which we used to eat free in Egypt, the cucumbers and the melons and the leeks and the onions and the garlic" (Num 11:5).

But we must ask, "What do these Old Testament laws have to do with healing for today?" As much as we might not understand the connection between the truth and healing, we should pay close attention because God is promising to heal, at least from some diseases. The truth communicates God's promises and will. Since God's intent is good, He offers protection from diseases. Those who conform their lives to God's Word, then, are protected.

In the end, though, it gets down to our personal lives. Would you carefully study and obey God's Word if it meant that you would be kept from disease?

> Curiously, would you do these things if you knew you would keep from cancer, heart disease, etc.?

It would follow logic that we would all do the things that God says in order to gain that extra level of protection, does it not? But people, as a whole, are not like that. They instead insist on disobeying the Lord and taking the risk. Consider the evident dangers of smoking. Do people choose to play Russian roulette with their cigarettes? Yes. We can go on and continue to add things to the list: divorce, drunkenness, overeating, etc. If anything, the human race has, by their foolish decisions proven that they are ensnared in the evil one's hand–caught, trapped, and dying (Eph 2:1-3).

God's not-so-special secret

So what brings healing? When you know Exodus 15:26, you know a very powerful secret–the promise of protection. The fulfillment of this promise is found when we know and do God's truth. If everyone started studying God's Word and obeying it, there would be a great reduction of diseases. Alone, we cannot change the world, though, so let's start smaller: what about you? Do you know God's Word? Do you obey it?

With man's tendency to sin, you would think that the Lord would give up and let him suffer.[1] But instead we find that

---

[1] The Lord did, in fact, do this in the flood but note that the Lord did not really start completely over, but worked through Noah and his family.

the opposite is true: He intercedes on our behalf. Jesus came, proclaiming God's Word with the hope that those who would hear and obey His words would gain eternal life. Jesus went a step further in John 3:36, "He who believes in the Son has eternal life; but he who does not obey the Son shall not see life, but the wrath of God abides on him."

In Exodus, God promised His people freedom from diseases if they obeyed His words. If they did not give heed to His Words, they would be more susceptible to disease. Here, in the Gospels, however, Jesus promises that those who obey Him will gain not just protection from a disease but life eternal! Without obedience, the wrath of God would rest on us.

Jesus first likens His words to God's—a quiet way of declaring His deity. They offer healing and life, even eternal life.

But instead of focusing on certain commands to obey, Jesus points out that life is secured only by faith in Him. This is because mankind lost the ability to obey the commands of God. Man is dying, but, if he believes in Jesus, he stands to gain two things: first, forgiveness, and second, eternal life. In other words, when we put our faith in Jesus, we are placing our dependence on Jesus, who lived uprightly, instead of on ourselves, who fail to live uprightly, time and time again.

While the Exodus commands will definitely help us avoid many diseases on earth, they won't help us in the end when death comes to our door. We need faith in Jesus in order to gain entrance into the land of health, that is, eternal life, where the curse of death is no more.

At one point Jesus spoke some strong words that offended some of His disciples, so they left. Turning to Peter, Jesus asked if he was going to leave Him too. Peter's answer is straightforward and exactly what we need to hear: "Simon Peter answered Him, "Lord, to whom shall we go? You have words of eternal life" (John 6:68-69).

God's words in Exodus 15:26 can lead to temporary health—those obedient to God's commands will not get the diseases so prevalent in the world. Jesus' words, however, are radically new and better as they offer eternal life rather than a way to simply avoid diseases. This is the reason spreading the gospel is so urgent: we are passing the cure for sin to those around us.

> "You have words of eternal life"
> (John 6:68).

#4 Study Questions

What cure does God give that will keep us from diseases (Ex 15:26)?

1. Does the Lord give us a cure for a disease in Ex 15:26? Explain.

2. What are the four instructions that He gives?

3. What is common between the first and third statements?

4. What is common between the second and fourth statements?

5. If you know something is good for you, do you always follow your advice? Explain.

6. Give an example, past or present, of your weakness where you gave in to your desires. List any consequence to doing that.

7. Curiously, would you follow these four instructions if you knew that it would prevent cancer, heart disease, etc.?

8. Why do many people doubt the value of God's Word to bring hope and life?

9. What will happen if anyone does not follow His advice?

10. What is the result if you follow these instructions in Exodus 15:26? Will you still die?

11. Read John 6:68-69. What is the result of following Jesus' words? Do you have this hope?

12. How would you answer the person who says that the Lord's commandments always keep us from our best?

The Lord Your Healer

Question #5

What does the truth of God's Word have to do with finding healing?

And He said, "If you will give earnest heed to the voice of the LORD your God, and do what is right in His sight, and give ear to His commandments, and keep all His statutes, I will put none of the diseases on you which I have put on the Egyptians; for I, the LORD, am your healer" (Ex 15:26).

The Lord our Creator has uncovered a powerful link here between His word and healing. Let us first note how He connects this healing with His words. The Lord tells us that if we obey these four things, none of the diseases out there in the world will touch our lives. In other words, God's words are spoken to protect and help God's people rather than to strip their freedoms from them, as is sometimes alleged. The devil has played too long with the lie that listening to God doesn't make a difference. The Devil tries to trick us into believing that God doesn't really care about what you do in private. We can fool ourselves all we want, but there's a bigger principle in operation.

Truth matters. Truth is freedom. It is just like Jesus said, "And you shall know the truth, and the truth shall make you free" (John 8:32). Many who are brought up in the church do not realize the blessings that they possess because they originate in a home where God's Word is kept and honored. It is easy to discard the truth of God when you are raised in a good home because it's difficult to see the connection between the keeping of God's word and those blessings, which, while temporary, are still good and should lead us to the Fount of eternal blessings. When we reject the truth of God, we will begin to see those blessings removed from our lives.

God's Word brings the desired blessings into our lives, just like the promise of protection from disease here in Exodus 15:26. His commands are good because they inherently bless us. But let's go back and ask the inevitable question, "What does truth have to do with me getting or not getting these diseases?" In order to answer this, I will list some diseases that are related to three kinds of sins and will show you specifically how they're related. Feel free to search the web and test this out. I have provided some documentation, but ample studies are available for further perusal.

Back in Moses' time, they were not able to verify God's Word the way our modern reports and statistics can. It now is very easy to see how, and if bias does not prevail, modern health apps will further prove, through a wider range of statistics, the connection between obedience to God's Word and healing. These facts will once again expose the evil one's lies, though you can be sure he will scamper about finding other lies to disguise the old ones. Remember our premise: obedience to God's commands brings a certain level of protection while disobedience opens the door for diseases to enter our lives. Our bodies were not made for certain lifestyles.

Study 1: Anger and Bitterness

Anger and an unforgiving spirit bring heart disease, broken relationships, and pride.

> Men who rate themselves as generally angry on questionnaires given early in life are, by the age of 55, three times more likely to have heart disease and six times more likely to have a heart attack (myocardial infarction), compared to other men." –The Johns Hopkins University study appears in today's (2002) Archives of Internal Medicine.[2]

Study 2: Worry and Anxiety

Out of Harvard Medical School, a study shows how worry and anxiety are at the roots of all sorts of diseases.

> Anxiety has now been implicated in several chronic physical illnesses, including heart disease, chronic respiratory disorders, and gastrointestinal conditions.[3]

---

[2] "Anger and Heart Disease" www.pcrm.org/health/medNews/anger-and-heart-disease

[3] "Anxiety and Physical Illness" www.health.harvard.edu/staying-healthy/anxiety_and_physical_illness

Study 3: Sexual Immorality

Sexual immorality leads to many sexually transmitted diseases (STDs) along with poverty and brokenness. The term "STD" connects sex outside of marriage with disease; if you want to avoid these diseases, it can be done by preserving your sexual purity for your marriage partner, future or present.

> Despite being a relatively small portion of the sexually active population, young people between the ages of 15 and 24 accounted for the highest rates of chlamydia and gonorrhea in 2014 and almost two thirds of all reported cases. Additionally, previous estimates suggest that young people in this age group acquire half of the estimated 20 million new STDs diagnosed each year.[4]

"In the sixties and seventies this relatively stable situation began to change."[5] Since the 1960s when premarital sex became more accepted, the number of common STDs jumped from 2 to around 25.[6] Yes, HIV and such infections can come from other sources such as used needles, but most come from disobedience to God in sexual immorality.

Is it worth debating? Hardly, as these things are now so common that the links between disobedience seen in sexual

---

[4] "Reported Cases of STDs on the Rise in the U.S." (Nov 2015) www.cdc.gov/nchhstp/newsroom/2015/std-surveillance-report-press-release.html

[5] https://www.probe.org/safe-sex-and-the-facts/

[6] http://www.faculty.fairfield.edu/faculty/hodgson/Courses/so142/premarital/premaritalTs.htm

immorality and sexually transmitted disease are readily apparent.

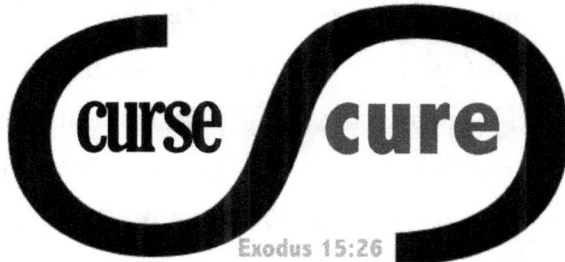

Exodus 15:26

Take the Sin out of curse and you end up with a cure.

The Lord has very carefully told us that we are not to vent our anger, worry, or live in fear, and to stay clear of all forms of sexual immorality both in the Old and New Testaments. The more promiscuous or addictive, the faster the diseases rush in.

What is your conclusion about these commands that God has given us, to keep us from disease? Following these commands lead us to best practices, and provides very good advice. Will they keep us from disease? Sure. The devil, however, attempts to confuse us with his lies, suggesting that God keeps the best from us by constraining us to His laws. And yet the opposite is true. God is the one who genuinely cares for us.

We cannot sufficiently emphasize the importance of obedience to the Lord. Whether you claim to be Buddhist or Christian, who will be protected? The one who conforms his or her life to God's Word. Who will suffer? Those who despise God's warning and wander from the clear path He's set out for us. His judgment will increase when we succumb to disobedience, though it is not to be considered a final punishment, for the great Day of Judgment is still coming.

Good nutrition is important, but it excludes the two key commands that God has provided for us so that we can have an extra level of protection from pain and suffering. Who loses if we choose to disobey? We do. God's Word is settled in heaven forever (Ps 119:89). Don't doubt it. Why is there a heroin crisis in America right now, even when people know overdosing is so easy and perilous? By their actions, they are trusting their own judgment rather than God's.

Signs of the curse generally increase with disobedience, which in turn serve as more severe warnings, pointing us back to repentance and obedience to God. Obedience restrains diseases from the cursed system under which we live. God's Word guides us to the truths we need to obey, leading us to trust in God's goodness and health.

Jesus comes at this issue from a different vantage point but concludes similarly to what is stated above.

> I am the door; if anyone enters through Me, he shall be saved, and shall go in and out, and find pasture. The thief comes only to steal, and kill, and destroy; I came that they might have life, and might have it abundantly (John 10:10).

So who are you going to trust? Jesus restated all these truths in the Sermon on the Mount (Mat 5-7). Now with many medical studies, we can validate God's Word as truth.

Obedience and devotion are related to health. Relax and enjoy seeking to know and follow the Lord's good words.

> "I am the door; if anyone enters through Me, he shall be saved, and shall go in and out, and find pasture. The thief comes only to steal, and kill, and destroy; I came that they might have life, and might have it abundantly" (John 10:10).

#5 Study Questions

What does the truth of God's Word have to do with finding healing?

1. If you were driving along a highway and saw a sign, "Caution: Bridge out ahead!" Would you slow down or stop?

2. Our culture is full of people who say that there is no absolute truth? Do you agree? Why or why not?

3. Read John 8:32. What does Jesus believe that the truth can do for us? What does that mean practically?

4. Where does God forbid or otherwise instruct His people not to be angry and harbor bitterness?

5. Which diseases are anger and bitterness linked to? (Feel free to reference the book or do your own search.)

6. Where does God forbid or otherwise instruct His people not to worry and be stressed out?

7. Which diseases are worry and anxiety linked to?

8. Where does God forbid or otherwise instruct His people not to conduct themselves in sexual immorality?

9. Which diseases are sexual immorality directly linked to?

10. Are you convinced that obedience leads to health and prevents all sorts of diseases? Explain.

11. Is premarital sex always wrong? Why do you say so?

12. Does Jesus promise to heal in John 10:10? What is life?

13. How will you briefly answer the person who dismisses God's Word as irrelevant?

The Lord Your Healer

Question #6

What does it mean that there's a larger purpose for healing than just the healing?

And He said, "If you will give earnest heed to the voice of the LORD your God, and do what is right in His sight, and give ear to His commandments, and keep all His statutes, I will put none of the diseases on you which I have put on the Egyptians; for I, the LORD, am your healer" (Ex 15:26).

Let's go back and take another look at Exodus 15:26. This verse claims more than we could ever imagine. Below is a diagram showing what this verse looks like. What do you see?

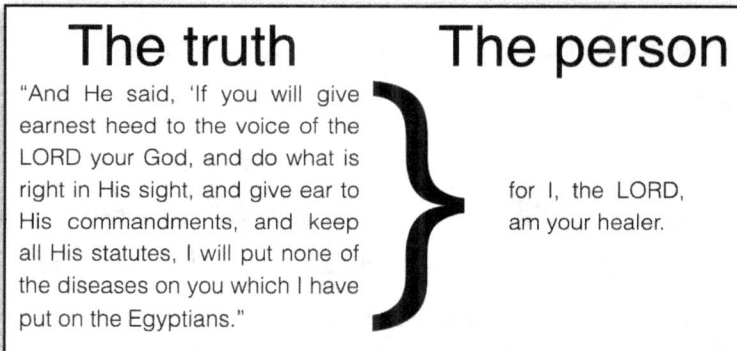

The truth	The person
"And He said, 'If you will give earnest heed to the voice of the LORD your God, and do what is right in His sight, and give ear to His commandments, and keep all His statutes, I will put none of the diseases on you which I have put on the Egyptians."	for I, the LORD, am your healer.

On the left we see the promise, that is, the four things that we need to do in order to have Jehovah God keep the diseases of the Egyptians from us. It simultaneously stands as a silent threat, though, because if the commands are not obeyed, the Egyptian diseases will come upon us.

Let's ask an important question: Where does healing come from? From obedience or from the Healer? It is easy to say that it comes out of obedience because it does. Obedience is what is requested. But why then is the 'for' statement–"for I, the LORD, am your healer"–included? The commandments and the healing lead to God. The Lord reminds us not to be entrapped by commandments or tradition, but to realize that their goal is a relationship with Him, which we know can only be found through Jesus Christ.

Goodness is found in the commandments because God is good. We find love and concern for the welfare of God's people because God is loving. There remains a challenge for each succeeding generation to use tradition to preserve the truth but also, as this verse reminds us, the responsibility to persistently point to the Person behind the truth. The Healer revealed His words of healing to us. When we pursue Him, we should realize we can trust and live in light of His presence (Ps 15:1-2).

For example, looking at the Old Testament temple from outside, you would have seen the priests, the temple walls, the garments, heard the law proclaimed and the singers sing of God. They were all existent and functioning at certain times, but they all exist there because of Yahweh God and His plan to dwell in the middle of His people. This exclusive focus on the religion became a major mistake with the religious Jews in Jesus' times. They were so fixed on the rules that they forgot about the one who gave the rules. This is similar to the problem people have in the Christian church, especially if they were brought up in the church culture. They equate knowledge and church experience with knowing God. This is a fatal mistake. Knowing one's Bible, though good, does not bring one into a relationship with God. This distinction is important for two reasons:

(1) No matter how much healing we might find now for our bodies and relationships, we will still die. Our ultimate healing is not found now, but in our new bodies, and in all the promises that will unfold at Christ's return. Temporary healing is insufficient. This is why the Lord told us where the healing comes from. He does not merely want to lead us to healthy lives, but ultimately He desires that we pursue Him.

(2) Our chief joy in life will not come from focusing on the commandments, as helpful as they are, but in knowing Christ and living in God's presence. The differences between the Old and New Testaments dramatically highlight this. In the Old Covenant, God lives hidden from His people, while in the New, God lives in His people through the Spirit of God. God's people become the temple! This is the same picture God gives us at the end of Revelation to teach us about eternity: we live in God's temple forever (Rev 21:1-4).

There is no healing apart from God. Healing is a means of grace working through humbling experiences that one may know and seek God's grace and discover the true Healer of life's final enemy, death itself through life eternal. Even if we find healing for another ten years like Hezekiah (Is 38:1-6), where will the body be after that?

Healing's ultimate purpose, then, is not to feel better but to know God more deeply. The commands, the truth of God, should open up our eyes to God's good and gracious heart. Of course, we all try to escape pain, discomfort, sickness, and disease, but we need to look beyond that need, no matter how desperate our situation.

No healthy person wants to meet God the Healer, because, in order to experience Him as such, one must enter some form of frailty to feel the touch of His healing hand. Yet, in actuality, we are all broken, diseased, and frail to some degree. The curse of our sin resides in us. The physical and relational problems we get only emphasize a truth we try to avoid, but it is, Jesus says, the starting point of the road to life—the first beatitude that leads to true blessings, "Blessed are the poor in spirit, for theirs is the kingdom of heaven" (Mat 5:3).

You might wonder about the kind of healing the Lord offers. I would suggest that you think of two things. First, try to think through some brokenness of heart, physical health, emotional trauma that you or another might be suffering. These troubles, then, form a call from the Healer, beckoning for that person to come, or if he knows the Lord, to come closer. Second, we can think of Jesus as the ultimate Healer.

He does not only save us from some physical problems, He also saves us from the devil, the world, and our own flesh, by giving us eternal life; He is the ultimate Healer, Jehovah Rophe. It is not the commands that care for us, though they bring healing, but the Healer Himself. He uses His words to direct us to Himself.

"Come to Me, all who are weary and heavy-
laden, and I will give you rest"
(Mat 11:28).

#6 Study Questions

What does it mean that there's a larger purpose for healing than just the healing?

1. According to Exodus 15:26, where does healing come from? Does healing come from obeying the command or from the Healer?

2. Do healing and help come from obedience to God's commands? Explain.

3. Does healing come from the Lord? Explain.

4. Why is healing so important to people?

5. Would you say that people are looking more for healing or for the Healer? Why so?

6. Why do you think the Lord included these last words, "for I, the Lord, am your healer"?

7. If you were the Healer, and people never said thanks for getting healing, what might you think?

8. Do you think people can be happy going to church and doing religion but never meeting the Savior? Discuss.

9. Why doesn't God just want us to obey these commands in Exodus 15:26 and live for another ten years, or does He have a greater goal?

10. What does it mean to meet or know God?

11. Read Matthew 11:28 and explain what Jesus promises and how you can gain it.

12. How might you briefly encourage a person to think beyond the healing and turn to the Healer?

The Lord Your Healer

Question #7

How are hospitals and physicians dependent on God's healing power?

And He said, "If you will give earnest heed to the voice of the LORD your God, and do what is right in His sight, and give ear to His commandments, and keep all His statutes, I will put none of the diseases on you which I have put on the Egyptians; for I, the LORD, am your healer" (Ex 15:26).

All hospitals and doctors are dependent on God's healing power. That is a bold statement, isn't it? With that one statement, we are claiming that hospitals, though equipped with the best medical equipment there is, are nothing without God's gracious extension of His merciful healing powers. This is what the Lord claims, "For I, the LORD, am your healer." (15:26)

Jehovah Rophe

אֲנִי יְהוָה רֹפְאֶךָ

The Lord's Name, Jehovah Rophe, is used here to provide deep insight into one aspect of who God is. He is the Healer.

The word used for 'healing' here means to 'mend by stitching' or, more figuratively, to cure.

The emphasis in this phrase is on the I: "for I, the Lord". In other words, Jehovah God claims the prerogative to heal as His.

Note the little word 'for' right before the Lord introduces His Name as Healer. This word demands that we go beyond merely looking at the commands the Lord gave us, and that we go beyond simply looking for healing. Something greater is happening, as was mentioned in the former chapter. The truth leads us to the person who spoke the truth just as the cure leads us to the Curer. God never intended that we strip His words of healing from Him. The power of the words are in Him–He is the Healer.

So let us more closely examine what the modern, secular society is claiming against the Lord.

The World's Lies	The Lord's Truths
Divorces morals from healing	Links morals with healing
Depends upon drugs to keep some health	Looks to Healer for healing
Thinks the best life is health and pleasure	Abundant life is found in Christ (Jn 10:10)
Deludes itself by thinking it can escape the curse	Peace (true healing) comes through faith in Christ

The Lord insists all healing stems from Himself, but secular society attempts to untie the knot linking truth with health. But it is not just the sick that need health; being under the curse, we are all constantly dependent upon the Lord for His merciful healing powers to sustain us. Because we feel young and vibrant, we are not on our knees often enough, pleading with and thanking Him. Even worse, we might even deny His Healing presence. Nevertheless, we must remain dependent upon Him and the measure of healing that He gives us. Through our actions and our words, we can protest His powers, but we are dependent upon his merciful acts of healing for every day we live.

Most of us probably look to drugs as the cure for our health issues, but why are we so quick to run to the pharmacy and ignore The Healer? I remember once using a chainsaw to cut down some small trees, and the next morning, my back was in a lot of pain. I carefully made my way to the medicine cabinet and took an Aleve without even once thinking of the Healer.

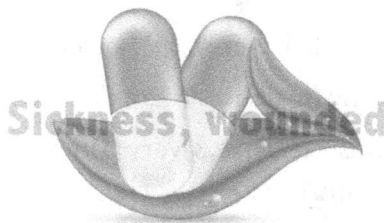

I had to confess my sin there. I put my hope in the medicine rather than the Healer. Instead, I should have reminded myself of how frail I am, that this body will soon die, but that

I am thankful for His merciful hand to hold me up each day. Then, if no healing had yet come to my back after seeking Him, use the pill and pray, "Lord take this and help restore my body to be able to carry out your will today." In this case, I would have sought Him and recognized His true place in my life.

Some people wonder if it is okay to take medicines. Besides the fact that we take far too many of them, and should seek out the source problem of why we need them (in case we have some kind of disobedience), we should take them moderately in faith, like James who was told to anoint with oil, the common medicinal oil back in that age. (Those in India still use many such medicinal oils.) "Is anyone among you sick? Let him call for the elders of the church, and let them pray over him, anointing him with oil in the name of the Lord" (James 5:14).

The world has become hedonistic, convinced that the best life is the one free to explore one's pleasures with the least amount of pain and cost possible. This summarizes life for many, especially the young, and they do this by using the days of God's extended mercy to worsen their situation. As noted elsewhere, the devil uses these deceptive conclusions to bring pain and misery. This is very different from Jesus the Healer who offers life.

Only in Jesus can you find true healing, not only for a time here on earth, but for eternity. Jesus offers eternal life and leaves the door open so that anyone can walk through into

His office where He personally counsels you as to your hopeless condition, but then takes off his white coat–exposing His marks on his hands and feet, points to how He carried your burden, disease, and death on the cross and promises to take you through into life eternal.

> I am the door; if anyone enters through
> Me, he shall be saved, and shall go in and
> out, and find pasture. The thief comes only
> to steal, and kill, and destroy; I came that
> they might have life, and might have it
> abundantly
> (John 10:10).

#7 Study Questions

How are hospitals and physicians dependent on God's healing power?

1. Do you agree that all hospitals and physicians are dependent on God's healing power? Explain.

2. How does the Lord describe Himself in Exodus 15:26?

3. Do you think these words convey the sense that the Lord believes He is the only Healer or just one of many? Explain.

4. Why do you think secular society is so insistent that they discover healing apart from God?

5. Give one example where people, ads, or movies suggest healing is not related to morals or obedience.

6. Is it wrong to only depend on drugs for getting better and forget God the Healer?

7. Think back on your life for an example of where you got help or took medicine and remembered God, as well as one time when you simply were looking for the healing.

8. Is it okay to take medicines? Discuss.

9. How does James 5:14 link oil (i.e., medicated oils) with the Lord?

10. Read John 10:10. What kind of life does Jesus offer? How can one gain it?

11. How healthy are you? Do you have life eternal? Explain your answer in light of Jesus' words in John 10:10.

12. What might you say to someone who arrogantly brags on the advances of modern science and health as if God has nothing to do with the healing process?

The Lord Your Healer

Question #8

Why do health plans bring more harm than good to people?

And He said, "If you will give earnest heed to the voice of the LORD your God, and do what is right in His sight, and give ear to His commandments, and keep all His statutes, I will put none of the diseases on you which I have put on the Egyptians; for I, the LORD, am your healer" (Ex 15:26).

The Lord claims to be the source of healing against all the diseases of the great nation of Egypt. His claim continues right into the modern age, even though the understanding of the body and healing processes has exponentially increased in recent years. But still, it is not medical devices, medicines, or prestigious doctors that heal but Jehovah Rophe. All of doctor's and researcher's wisdom comes from discovering how God made the body and the relationships within that body that are necessary for proper function. Note these powerful words:

"And He said, 'If you will', then He will ...put none of the diseases on you." It is critical that we quickly discern the problems, personal and societal, stemming from denying the connection between health and the truth of God's word. The truth is the facts, which remains impervious to what we think of it. No matter what we think about the words of protection in Exodus 15, the truth still connects our disobedient behaviors with diseases. One doctor personally said to me that more than 60% of today's diseases result from what people call unhealthy choices.

The Lord has provided the connection between our behavior and disease so that we would turn away from evil (i.e. disobedience) and do what is right and good. Remember, His commands and words bring life. Note God's good intention:

> So that you and your son and your grandson might fear the LORD your God, to keep all His statutes and His commandments, which I command you, all the days of your life, and that your days may be prolonged (Deut 6:2).

> For the commandment is a lamp, and the teaching is light; and reproofs for discipline are the way of life (Prov 6:23).

> And I know that His commandment is eternal life; therefore the things I speak, I speak just as the Father has told Me (John 12:50).

With this introduction, let us get back to evaluating health insurance plans, whether private or national. My assessment is that as long as people do not need to personally, upfront, pay the cost of their mistakes, they will not learn from them, change, and get better. Health insurance programs, as a whole, cover up the sins of some and distribute the cost to the rest. As long as this happens, people have little motivation to improve their behavior. They figure, ridiculously so, that they will be one of the individuals that does better than the rest. They know that if disease crops up, their plan will cover it.

And so, while their behavior is something they could change, they don't. Everyone pays for that person's sinful choices. What if we had people who smoke more than a pack a month pay upfront, say $100 extra every month.[7] Only then, perhaps, would they start to see the pain of their decisions. Health insurance plans now–with rare exclusions–induce illness and disease by covering many different items, increasing people's boldness in making foolish and immoral decisions. These plans do not actually care for people; instead, they promote bad health and even reward it.

The most obvious is abortion. Here in the USA, about one million people are killed every year. Because someone else pays and the government says okay, young mothers and fathers think it an option to kill their own child. And so the list goes on: ongoing anxiety, drug addictions, etc. As long as the costs are all covered easily, people will not be willing to

---

[7] A tax does not bring enough sting nor emphasize the seriousness of their ill choices. Excluding lung treatment for smokers from the plan, for example, will highlight this link and so does an extra cost (if they want lung cancer treatment to be covered), both providing extra motivation to stop smoking.

change what they do to achieve better health overall, nor will they seek the Healer.

This is the reason it is imprudent to put the burden of medical treatment for obviously poor choices on those in a joint plan rather than penalizing the individual. Why have everyone pay for the sinful choices of others? No one will take responsibility and change their behavior for good because medical plans cover up the connection between immorality, disease, and cost, and when the burden of consequence is lifted, it takes away any motivation to make the healthiest choices. What happens as a result is that health plans become very expensive and less attention is focused on diseases that do not originate with poor choices.[8]

If the doctor told you to take a pill and follow directions, would you follow them? Most of us would. Your Healer is beckoning you to follow His cure so that things might be well with you. God, your Healer, offers not only a temporary cure but an eternal one if we would but listen and follow Him. May we all listen to Him! What a wonderful improvement our lives would see! But most importantly, we would again believe that God genuinely wants our best.

> "But whoever drinks of the water that I
> shall give him shall never thirst; but the
> water that I shall give him shall become in
> him a well of water springing up to eternal
> life" (John 4:14).

---

[8] Consider the foolishness of long lines at emergency rooms in the big cities.

#8 Study Questions

Why do health plans bring more harm than good to people?

1. Although medical research has exponentially increased in the last decade, including studies on the DNA, would you still say the Lord is the Healer?

2. What percentage of diseases would you estimate come from 'unhealthy' choices?

3. What percentage of the medical health budget covers these unhealthy choices?

4. Why does the Lord allow a disease to crop up when people disobey Him?

5. How do health plans disguise the link between sinful choices and diseases? How could it be made clearer?

6. Do you think if people had to contribute an extra $20 to each package of cigarettes that would later be used to treat their lung cancer that this would help form the connection between their choices and the results?

7. What might happen if health plans only covered those diseases and treatments not directly related to one's sinful choices?

8. I claim that governments and plans do not have the best interests of the people in mind when using health plans without qualification. Do you agree? Explain.

9. Read John 4:14. How does the healing that hospitals and drugs offer compare to Jesus' offer? Explain.

10. How might you briefly answer someone that adamantly states that national health insurance is the only way?

The Lord Your Healer

Question #9

Is all sickness related to my personal sin?

And He said, "If you will give earnest heed to the voice of the LORD your God, and do what is right in His sight, and give ear to His commandments, and keep all His statutes, I will put none of the diseases on you which I have put on the Egyptians; for I, the LORD, am your healer" (Ex 15:26).

If you have been paying close attention to this study, you are more than likely itching to ask this question. Or, perhaps, a question like, "How does my personal sin affect my health?" We will take a look at this question and clarify the truth that will keep us from Satan's deceit, and more importantly, will allow the Words of God to lead us deeper into truth and our trust in God.

As the question stands, we might feel like a big failure once we look at this question. When looking at these verses, it's easy to conclude that all our pain and brokenness are due to our personal sins. Many of them, admittedly, might be so. This shallow understanding ends up with some Christians mistakingly–though in earnest good intention–saying, "Since we all sin, including me, I cannot judge the wrongness of another's choices." We agree we all stand on the side of the guilty, but does God want us to broadcast Satan's deceitful lies or the gospel? Should we suggest that the love of God obliterates judgment regardless of our response to the Healer? Personal sin should not ever be considered inconsequential.

Satan can maliciously take this wrong conclusion (all my pain is due to my personal sin) and cause many a believer to feel horribly guilty, sometimes to the point of giving up. The truth is, they are guilty and deserve judgment, but they forget the redeeming work of Christ. Some believers prone to anxiety can end up with guilt plaguing their minds, leading them into a depressed life. Satan feeds these people wrong conclusions, leaving them spiritually crippled.

The Lord never says that there is a one hundred percent connection with our personal sin and our health situation. There is a better way of looking at our situation, whether you're a believer or not. We can prove this simply by looking at Job, who was a righteous man and suffered greatly, even though He hadn't done anything wrong to deserve it. God actually favored him (Job 1:8)! For us to conclude that every pimple and rash is related to some specific sin of ours becomes unhelpful and far from the truth. Satan uses these false conclusions to get people to condemn themselves. "I have a fever. Oh, what did I do wrong?" This is not a healthy approach to our lives. Satan's name means 'accuser' because he persistently wants to bring our sins and guilt down upon our heads. This kind of thinking does not lead to salvation, and worse, some people, even after hearing the gospel, will say, "I am not good enough." What they really mean, thanks to Satan's input, "I am too bad to be saved." By believing this lie, they put themselves in a pit.

So let's return to the question, "What is the relationship between my sin, health, and choices?" On the one hand, diseases are related to our personal choices. Anger can bring on heart disease, while sexual immorality spreads STDs. But in reality, our physical and relational problems go far beyond this.

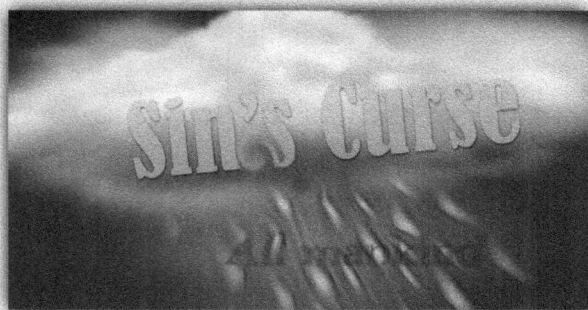

We start, not with our personal sins, but by acknowledging that all of mankind lives under the general curse of sickness, suffering, and pain, all of which leads to death. Even without consideration of our personal sins, we will still face troublesome physical ailments that are not related to any particular sins but are due to bearing up under the harsh, demanding general curse of death. That was the result of our forefather's disobedience to God.

Within that greater context, then, we have our own personal choices that can, if in agreement with God's Word, shelter us from the harshness of the curse, or contrariwise, accelerate the pain and suffering that we experience on earth. Personal sin habits create easy access, like broken down doors, for the curse's assailing storm to strike us where we are vulnerable.

Is all sickness related to my personal sin? No, but it is related to sin. Just because judgment is coming, we shouldn't consider speeding up the process by our personal sinful choices.

Obedience to God's Word brings rewards that are seen in the lives of godly people who are passing enjoyable lives on earth. Our goal is not an easy life, however, for our hope is placed beyond the reach of the devastating curse. Our preoccupation, instead, is how can we offer this good news of forgiveness of sin and eternal life through Jesus to others before the final judgment.

> "And there shall no longer be any curse;
> and the throne of God and of the Lamb
> shall be in it, and His bond-servants shall
> serve Him" (Rev 22:3).

#9 Study Questions

Is all sickness related to my personal sin?

1. Do all your health problems stem from your personal sin? Explain.

2. Why is it wrong to refuse to condemn sin by admitting that we are sinners too? What is a better response?

3. Why does Satan suggest that people are guilty and can't do any good?

4. How does Job 1:8 show that there is not a one hundred percent direct correlation between sin and suffering?

5. Is anyone too bad to be saved?

6. Is anyone too good not to be judged?

7. How does the general curse (Gen 3) relate to our imperfect health?

8. How do our personal choices and situations relate to other diseases or sicknesses that we might get?

9. Read Revelation 22:3. What is the curse? What will happen to it? How so?

10. What might you briefly say to those who seem to have given up hope on themselves because of their many wrongs?

The Lord Your Healer

Question #10

How can health become a block to a person knowing and discovering God?

And He said, "If you will give earnest heed to the voice of the LORD your God, and do what is right in His sight, and give ear to His commandments, and keep all His statutes, I will put none of the diseases on you which I have put on the Egyptians; for I, the LORD, am your healer" (Ex 15:26).

It seems to be a bit contrary to suggest that health can block the path to know and experience God our Healer, but I want to argue that it definitely can. This is one reason, I believe, that in the above verse the word 'for' is included. People can find healing by obeying the Lord, growing up in a good Christian family or a culture where they respect parents. Paul quotes one of the ten commandments that has a promise. "Children, obey your parents in the Lord, for this is right. Honor your father and mother (which is the first commandment with a promise), that it may be well with you, and that you may live long on the earth" (Eph 6:1-3; Deut 5:16).

Do you see the pattern? Obedience brings blessing. The more a society esteems respect for their parents, the better the society will be, and of course, the less sin, trouble, and suffering will occur. This can be proven by tracing the backgrounds of juvenile delinquents. A large number of these juvenile delinquents come from fatherless homes, which often means the presence of sexual immorality, selfishness, and unfaithfulness or disobedience.[9]

You would think that everyone would run in obedience to gain a better life, but there's a tragic misunderstanding that creates a blockage. Children in good homes and cultures grow up and take the joy of their families as normal and tend to consider God to be an irrelevant factor of their good lives. It is like someone thinking the computer can run without the processor. What a horrible mistake the young make! Whenever the link between blessing and obedience is broken, forgotten, or otherwise considered to be irrelevant, problems ensue. Right now, our society is at the end of one of these moments. It does not mean everyone is as bad as they could be, but that there is little good culture that encourages proper behavior and obedience to God (even when that culture doesn't know that God is behind it). Even when God is recognized, He is still often seen as an unwanted accessory.

---

[9] "Statistics on Fatherless Children in America" http://fatherhood.about.com/od/fathersrights/a/fatherless_children.htm

This is nothing new, of course. God has, numerous times before, warned us of disregarding Him. He does it here in Exodus 15:26 by claiming that He is behind all healing. The Lord painfully shows us that healing, life, and peace all are connected to Him—not just some culture or religious custom. "Be careful to listen to all these words which I command you, so that it may be well with you and your sons after you forever, for you will be doing what is good and right in the sight of the Lord your God" (Deut 12:28). Right after the Ten Commandments are given in Deuteronomy 5, a serious warning is stated several times for effect regarding the danger of forgetfulness.

> Then it shall come about when the Lord your God brings you into the land which He swore to your fathers, Abraham, Isaac and Jacob, to give you, great and splendid cities which you did not build, and houses full of all good things which you did not fill, and hewn cisterns which you did not dig, vineyards and olive trees which you did not plant, and you eat and are satisfied, **then watch yourself, that you do not forget the Lord** who brought you from the land of Egypt, out of the house of slavery. You shall fear only the Lord your God; and you shall worship Him and swear by His name (Dt 6:10-13).

Do you see the pattern? God brings help and healing, His people are blessed, then the people become forgetful of this connection between God's blessing and obedience, so they put their hearts on other things and increasingly harsh signs

connected to the curse break out upon them Deut
31:16-18).

One of these blessings is healing, which the Lord confidently
states again, "The Lord will remove from you all sickness; and
He will not put on you any of the harmful diseases of Egypt
which you have known, but He will lay them on all who hate
you" (Deut 7:15).

The warning, earlier seen in chapter 6, is repeated in chapter
8. The Lord knows how easily mankind is disoriented by
blessings:

> Beware that you do not forget the Lord your God by
> not keeping His commandments and His ordinances
> and His statutes which I am commanding you today;
> otherwise, when you have eaten and are satisfied, and
> have built good houses and lived in them, and when
> your herds and your flocks multiply, and your silver
> and gold multiply, and all that you have multiplies,
> then your heart will become proud and you will forget
> the Lord your God who brought you out from the land
> of Egypt, out of the house of slavery (Deut 8:11-14).

Of course, we respond to God, "We know. You don't have to
treat us as kids and repeat yourself!" But the problem is that
this tendency to forget God when all is going well is a huge
problem for every one of us. God's point of bringing healing
and other blessings upon our lives is to show us how
obedience brings blessings to our lives and, in fact, brings us
to God Himself—our true Healer.

Jesus saw this same tendency of looking for blessings rather than God in the lives of His disciples. "Jesus answered them and said, "Truly, truly, I say to you, you seek Me, not because you saw signs, but because you ate of the loaves, and were filled. Do not work for the food which perishes, but for the food which endures to eternal life, which the Son of Man shall give to you, for on Him the Father, even God, has set His seal" (John 6:26-27).

Healing, along with other blessings, can at times, become our chief focus. When it is our chief focus, it becomes a stumbling block. We either take the healing and forget the Lord, much like nine of the ten lepers, or later on, let our hearts' affection for God wane. Jesus rightly spurs us onward:

> "Do not work for the food which perishes,
> but for the food which
> endures to eternal life."
> (John 6:27).

#10 Study Questions

How can health become a block to a person knowing
and discovering God?

1. In review, how does Exodus 15:26 connect obedience,
   healing, and the Healer?

2. What does God offer those who obey their parents (Eph
   6:1-3; Deut 5:16)?

3. What will happen to those who do not obey and respect
   their parents?

4. How does the statistics regarding juvenile delinquents
   back up the truth behind this promise?

5. How does a conforming culture or family that
   encourages obedience to parents become a blessed and
   successful one?

6. A good life comes from good choices. Why is it that
   young people sometimes are not so convinced?

7. If people are not convinced of the connection between
   obedience and blessings, what might they do? (This is
   what happened in the 1960s in America.)

8. Right after Deuteronomy 5 where the Ten Commandments were given, God brought a warning. Read Deuteronomy 6:10-13 and state what God warns them of?

9. Do you think that this warning is applicable to us too? How so?

10. Explain the pattern from Deuteronomy 6:10-18 here. Where are you in this process?

11. Read John 6:27. Which kind of food is more important? How does this relate to the above discussion?

12. Who might you briefly warn a friend or child that they should not take their blessings and measure of healing for granted?

The Lord Your Healer

Question #11

How is healing an illustration of the Gospel?

And He said, "If you will give earnest heed to the voice of the LORD your God, and do what is right in His sight, and give ear to His commandments, and keep all His statutes, I will put none of the diseases on you which I have put on the Egyptians; for I, the LORD, am your healer" (Ex 15:26).

People love miracle workers, but physical healing is not our final answer. Those healed will still die! Healing, then, serves as a sign pointing to something greater, and as such, it becomes an illustration of salvation. While Exodus 15:26 refers exclusively to shielding those obedient to God's Word from physical diseases, salvation rescues the believers from spiritual death for eternal life. Although we have throughout this book linked healing with certain gospel truths, we have not shown how health fully illustrates salvation in the gospel, something we will now do.

Unlike some religions like Hinduism and Buddhism, where they see death as a means to escape the material body connected to sin for a spiritual salvation, the Bible teaches us very differently. Salvation in the scriptures is described as the rescuing of the body and soul from God's judgment, which is accomplished in death (Gen 3:3).

John 3:36 says "the wrath of God abides on us." This wrath is the same as God's just sentence waiting to be fully carried out because of Adam's sin in the Garden of Eden. As our representative of all mankind, Adam failed the test by eating the forbidden fruit, so sin terribly affected all of us (Gen 3:1-11). The Apostle Paul goes on in detail connecting our lives and situations with Adam's fall from God's grace. "Therefore, just as through one man sin entered into the world, and death through sin, and so death spread to all men, because all sinned" (Rom 5:12). Somewhere in there, we are all included, as Adam's descendants.[10]

God's people are delivered from this curse by Jesus' willingness to die on our behalf. He died for us. This is the significance of the cross. There were many people in that day being killed on crosses as a form of execution. Jesus, however, did no wrong but took the judgment of His people on Himself and in so doing, gave us His righteousness. By satisfying God's wrath,

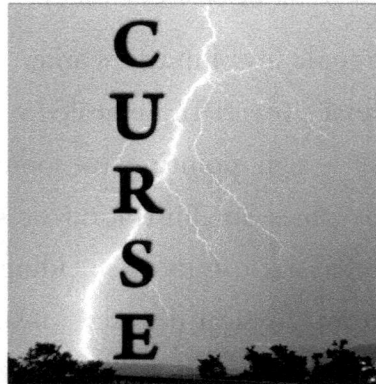

---

[10] Those who espouse evolution often disregard the implications of the fall by denying a fully mature and upright man's disobedience before God. Jesus, however, believed in a literal Adam and Eve (Mat 19:4-5).

Jesus set us free from the judgment. (The word propitiation, used four times in the scriptures, declares this very fact.)

Healing, then, only holds off death's curse from our lives, but Jesus' death on the cross actually fully satisfies God's judgment and removes the curse from us, bringing us from darkness into light. "I have come as light into the world, that everyone who believes in Me may not remain in darkness" (John 12:46).

But the removal of the curse from us, though great, is only part of the deliverance. A new faith in Christ's work on the cross also brings new life, which leads to eternal life because it keeps on going. This new life, however, finds its ultimate hope in the resurrection of the body, which is similar to Jesus' resurrected body. So physical healing is very temporary and limited. After all, healing is only needed for a decaying body. Cells die every day. Healing is only temporary, but eternal life promises an ongoing, vibrant new body that can live fully in God's presence. Healing, again, points to God's mercy, but what God gives us is not only mercy in holding back His wrath upon us but also mercy in greatly blessing us with eternal life.

> "So that, as sin reigned in death, even so grace would reign through righteousness to eternal life through Jesus Christ our Lord" (Rom 5:21).

Healing, then, is a temporary extension of life to mankind, and while that is good, we should focus on God's offer of eternal life. With most people now living into their 70's and 80's, the opportunity to experience temporary healing and to find eternal life is extended. At a certain point in history, though, the curse like a vicious thunderstorm, waits for its time to break over our heads. And yet, even in those breaking storms, God's mercy, through healing, keeps our sick-prone bodies alive.

History, then, is not only an extension of our opportunity to experience God's mercy, but for God, within that designated time frame to send His Son into the world to be born, die, and be resurrected, thus giving those who believe in God's promised One, to find life eternal. That is right, not just temporary healing to relieve us from a disease but full healing from sin's curse.

Repentance is an important part of salvation because it describes the discovery of our personal sin and rebellion, recognizes ourselves as in the wrong, and in response seeks a way out of God's judgment. And faith plays an important role in repentance. We see how Jesus graciously came and died to take our burden from us. Our hearts ought to be overwhelmed! Just like a person who has been healed from a disease goes around telling everyone the story, so we ought to love to share how we were spiritually healed.

People often get confounded wondering how a loving God can tolerate the existence of hell. God could have designed the world that way, but He wanted to show the awesomeness of His mercy to us. God doesn't overlook our sinfulness, but suffered for us. This work on the cross shows the extreme mercy and love of God.

> "For even the Son of Man did not come to
> be served, but to serve, and to give His life
> a ransom for many"
> (Mark 10:45).

#11 Study Questions

How is healing an illustration of the Gospel?

1. How does Exodus 15:26 say that we can gain a measure of protection from disease?

2. Whose words are we to follow?

3. Why are the Lord's words so important compared to others?

4. What happened when Adam disobeyed God's words (Genesis 3:3)? Look at Romans 5:12 and describe how this affected everybody.

5. How does this curse on mankind relate to God's personal handling of us (John 3:36)?

6. Do you think if we try to be good that things will get better? Explain.

7. How does Romans 5:12 point to a way out from under the curse?

8. Explain how healing is linked to life and death linked to the curse.

9. Why does God not offer permanent healing now for believers?

10. Why did God send His only Son, Jesus Christ, to die for the sins of His people (Mark 10:45)?

11. Do you believe the Gospel and have eternal life?

   • If so, share the Gospel, or part of it, with another person.

   • If not, identify what part you are hesitant over believing. Consider believing now!

The Lord Your Healer

Question #12

So how should I treat the pain, diseases, and broken relationships that I face?

And He said, "If you will give earnest heed to the voice of the LORD your God, and do what is right in His sight, and give ear to His commandments, and keep all His statutes, I will put none of the diseases on you which I have put on the Egyptians; for I, the LORD, am your healer" (Ex 15:26).

As we contemplate our painful lives in tandem with the amount of healing necessary for restoration, let us attempt to provide an answer on how to personally face pain and suffering in our daily lives. It is not uncommon to get sick, suffer a sprain, get a sore throat, or discover a disease deeply embedded in your body. Even children get sick, but they more than often pop right back to full health. The common adage among adults is, "I'm getting older." This, of course, hints at an increase in the number of health problems that you'll encounter as you get older. Does this Exodus verse offer any guidance for us?

There are several factors that we need to be attentive to when we get sick. Let me identify them.

The Lord is the only Healer. We can be grateful for medications, doctors, nurses, and hospitals, but we also much remember that we are not subject to them as if they are the only hope we have. Jesus healed many and the He can heal us too. Although our situation might be permanent according to doctors, it also might not be. Keep your focus on the Lord your Healer rather than the method of treatment. The advice, drugs, and treatment are only meant to assist you in the healing process. No doctor 'heals' but only leads you to the path where healing in the Lord's hands can be found.

Our goal, then, should be bigger than just being healed. Healing is only a means to better know the Healer. If we are healed, go home, and never get closer to God, then we should consider ourselves missing the whole point of the exercise.

We should not be afraid of our pains and physical distresses—though they be so troublesome and even limiting. When you find yourself calling 911 for an ambulance, trust God with the whole situation through a quick prayer. We can rightly look to Him for healing, even while seeing many doctors, visiting hospitals, and undergoing tests.

We can attentively (or have someone help us) oversee what medication we are taking and the procedures being recommended. Second opinions are definitely recommended for anything half-serious because advice comes from different experiences. Pray without ceasing.

Reflect on your own personal life. What has God created you for? What has He so far done through your life? What does

He yet want to do? When our health goes, we are weak and vulnerable, but this is exactly what we need in order to humbly reconsider our past choices. Sometimes the Healer points out past sins that we need to confess. At other times, people will share about Jesus and the cross, and it will become clear to you like never before. There are no limits to what God can do through your weaknesses and vulnerabilities. Believe on Him and find eternal life.

As His child, never consider these times to be unnecessary, but as a time God is reshaping you, the way you think, the way you function, etc.

Let me share a personal story from 2013. When in Nepal on one of my trips training pastors, I was packing up and readying to go back to my home after I had conducted all the training sessions for the Christian workers. Somehow, I pulled my back so that I was in excruciating pain no matter what position I was in. That was the morning of a very long trip, over 24 hours, to return home. I couldn't sit down and I couldn't stand up. But there I was trying to manage my luggage. I prayed a lot during that time. I did not complain (that I remember) but accepted this reminder of my frailty.

Did I know what spiritual battle the Lord was preparing me for? No, but I knew I could trust Him. Was He testing me? Of course. I wanted to stay faithful. There were 6 hours before my fast (that I had already voluntarily started) would end, so I chose to refrain from medication. I did what I could, trying to find positions and exercises that would alleviate the pain at least a little.

I could trust my Lord with this slowing down of my schedule, with the extra pain, and sought to meet Him more. I began to understand even more significantly how much I needed my Savior. He became so dear to me. I was not complaining, but accepted my limitations as necessary, and I wasted no time in stepping closer to Him.

So, on the one hand, I used this time to draw closer to Him, but on the other, I also tried to alleviate the pain. I had the other pastors pray for me before sending me off. I suffered quite a bit before getting better, but it was a reminder that my ministry and life itself was in His hands. That could have been the last mission trip for me as far as I knew.

In trying to cope with the pain on my way home, I went go through many humbling experiences. At one check point, I had to lift my bag from the floor onto the inspection table. I looked at the soldier who just stared at me waiting. I could pick it up, but only with great pain, I bent my knees and descended to the floor like an elevator, pulling the bag against me, and straightened up, extending the bag out like a robot. I put it back the same way. How far would the Lord test me? I didn't know, but I resolved to be faithful and trust Him the Healer. Yes, later, I could take a pain reliever, and that made sitting possible on the flight back, but I would not take my eyes off Him.

The Lord is the Healer; He is Jehovah Rophe. He alone is the means by which we depend on for wellness and we can trust Him for endurance through the rough times. We are all partaking in His healing every day, otherwise, we would die. But it is good to use our times of brokenness to refresh our acquaintance with Him so that we never forget how much He cares for us, and so that we stay on track with the mission He has assigned us.

Our major goal in life is not to get through life with the least pain possible, but to know and exalt our God despite the extremity of our tests. He is, after all, our Savior, which is another name for Super Healer. We are in His hands, secured under His protection, awaiting for the full healing, the day we cast off these diseased bodies and turn them in for a new resurrected body, to live with Him forever. If you desire healing now, shouldn't you want healing forever? And if you love health, should you not adore the Healer?

> "Who are protected by the power of God
> through faith for a salvation ready to be
> revealed in the last time"
> (1 Peter 1:5).

#12 Study Questions

So how should I treat the pain, diseases, and broken relationships that I face?

1. Even though we might have eternal life through faith in Christ, we still suffer pains, sicknesses, and fevers. List a few of your symptoms.

2. Should we avoid drugs, doctors, and hospitals, or is it a show of lack of trust in God our Healer? Explain.

3. What does it mean by: "No doctor heals"? Do you agree?

4. Is it wrong to want to feel better? Explain.

5. How should we think about God when getting a cold or calling emergency for help?

6. Why can we trust God for giving us the measure of health we need to carry out the work He has for us?

7. Does God still love us even when we face excruciating pain? How do we know this?

8. How should we treat those times when we are called to slow down due to sickness or pain? Should we think of it positively or negatively? Why?

9. If the Lord is the Healer, why does He sometimes hold back healing from me or others?

10. What does 1 Peter 1:5 say that will protect our faith while being tested? Can you share an illustration where you saw this working out?

11. How might you briefly encourage a believer to positively look upon his sickness rather than in bitterness?

The Lord Your Healer

Question #13

How should I or others face the possibility of death through sickness?

And He said, "If you will give earnest heed to the voice of the LORD your God, and do what is right in His sight, and give ear to His commandments, and keep all His statutes, I will put none of the diseases on you which I have put on the Egyptians; for I, the LORD, am your healer" (Ex 15:26).

The Lord tells us in Exodus 15:26 that when we obey Him, we will not suffer diseases as the world experiences. But, all of a sudden, my wife is in the emergency room. How should she respond? As her husband and as a minister of the Gospel, how do I respond? Lots of questions pop up: "Will she live?" "What if she doesn't return to full health?" "Can I afford the treatment? If so, for how long?" "Can the children manage?" "How will this affect my work?" The Lord has revealed to us the course of avoiding many diseases, but sickness and disease are still hunting us down until our bodies succumb to death's final stab.

In the spring of 2014, my wife Linda started having a difficult time climbing steps. One day as we were heading out for our weekly date, she suggested I should first take her to the doctor's office. Upon examining her, the doctor immediately sensed something was wrong and sent her to the emergency room. (So much for our date!) There she was found to have a disease: congestive heart failure (CHF), where her heart was functioning only at about 35%. Death was near to her. Somehow her heart got weak, big, and ineffective. There was no known cause.

In Linda's case, she did get heart disease. Although we could not point to the particular cause of the disease, we kept seeking the Healer Himself. We examined our lives for any known sin but could not pinpoint any.[11] We had others from around the world join us in prayer for her. In this case, there was no cure-all medicine or procedure. In other words, there wasn't much the doctors could do. The medicine that was given to her would only slow down her heart, thus making her feel crummy, weak, and tired, and forcefully slowed down her lifestyle. This is rather hard to do when you have had eight children, four of which were still at home, as well as some grandchildren nearby! Linda, however, did see the doctor and, according to the doctor's advice, went through some

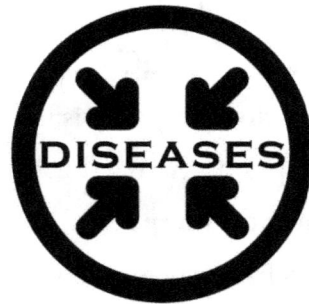

---

[11] This free extended Bible study can deepen your acquaintance with this important James 5 passage. www.foundationsforfreedom.net/References/NT/Others/James/James5_14-18_Questions.html

testing, and later took her prescribed medications after staying a number of days in the hospital.

There are some that see medication as an enemy to the faith. They can be, but as James says, we can use such agents, like medicinal oils, to assist in healing (James 5:13-16). Carefully used together with seeking the Healer, God can and does grant healing.

But we also should be cautious against the fatalist mentality, which sees disease as the final word. "If I get the disease, then I will not fight it." Sometimes this happens on a death bed. When we know it is time to go because of some extensive deterioration of health, then it is proper to get ready to see the Lord. God, however, is on our side to fight against sickness and death. Hezekiah was not chastised when seeking for healing (Isaiah 38), nor were the many who came to Jesus for healing. Jesus healed them. It follows, then, that we ought to see disease and sickness, not as a sign to give up to death, but to better pursue the Healer. We need to use our faith to approach Him as our Healer. Getting people to pray with us for my wife, taking medicine, and observing a modified diet were all steps in an attempt to restore her, but we needed to remember that the methodology should never interfere with the call to seek the Healer Himself.

There is, in America, the huge problem of cost. Each family needs to consider the financial cost to any attempted method of treatment. Although healing is what we should seek, the costs must be weighed against the risks and hopes. I remember meeting two little orphaned children in Nigeria and wondering what happened to their parents; I found out that their parents had not had money for antibiotic pills and promptly died. On the other hand, we see some families going seriously into debt for an elderly parent, and, though trying to be respectful, they are not being very wise. When the parent dies, the family will lose everything under the crushing debt. As much as we esteem life, falling into severe debt is not right either.[12]

What if God didn't heal my wife? As her husband, I had to prepare myself for the 'What ifs.' "What if she could only operate at 50% for the rest of her life?" "What if the doctors recommend a heart transplant?" I need to prepare myself, my family, my hopes, and my ministry by giving them to God and praying seriously about them.

A doctor's advice and treatment are sometimes wrong, such as in testing the health of a child before it is born. They might count it as routine, but it puts a burden on the hopeful parents if they hear the baby has some disease or problem. We should not put the child to death because of a potential health problem but live under God's mercy as He wills. I have heard how parents in such a case went ahead with the baby and found out the baby was perfectly healthy. Why have the test?

---

[12] Hospitals in America are not fair in that they do not tell you upfront how much a treatment will cost. Instead of one signature for full treatment, they should be, in my view, accountable to pay your bill unless they give you an estimate of the costs.

Jesus performed many miracles to establish that He is to be believed in as the Savior, and in keeping, John was quite clear on his purpose in writing, "But these have been written that you may believe that Jesus is the Christ, the Son of God; and that believing you may have life in His name" (John 20:31). There it is again, the word 'life.' It is a word I have had a hard time trying to grasp over the years. Why did He promise life? The meaning of this word has become much clearer to me in recent years. Life is offered to those who are perishing. Death has claimed us, but Jesus offers eternal life to us. It will not come naturally, with meditative exercises, or even by eating organic foods. Our life is our opportunity to find not temporary healing to get us out of a bout with death, but life eternal through Jesus Christ, a place where we will live in Jehovah Rophe's presence forever.

Exodus 15:26 reminds us that all sickness, pain, and suffering that is found in things like poor relationships become a call to enter the presence of the Healer, Jehovah Rophe. We might go to the doctor's and visit the hospital, but we must chiefly look for a visit from Jehovah Rophe. I am not saying that we should at all be ungrateful for kind and experienced doctors, but that true healing comes not from the procedures themselves but from the Healer. I am not speaking of a mystical encounter that brings miraculous healing, but opportunities to reflect on our lives and place our lives into His hands. Many people do not know the Lord. They might be religious, but they do not know the Lord as Healer and Savior. The Lord uses all things, including fatal diseases, to shake our lives that we might turn and find Him. Such times are certainly the times to hear and believe the Gospel of Jesus. Opportunities to seek healing from sickness are always reminders to seek Life Himself.

Somehow, with the prayers around the world for Linda, God healed her. The doctor said that healing doesn't usually happen in such cases, and more typically she would have needed a heart transplant. But here she is, two years later, off of all heart medication and no restrictions on her diet. Shortly after hearing of her healing, short of one year of discovering the problem, the two of us went off to speak at a parenting seminar in Taiwan and a marriage seminar in Burma (Myanmar). God's miraculous healing extended our opportunities to serve Him!

Jesus appeared in His resurrected body, and Thomas, seeing the holes in Jesus' hands, humbly remarked to Him, "My Lord and my God" (John 20:27-28)! Jesus brought the conversation to another level when He replied, "Because you have seen Me, have you believed? Blessed are they who did not see, and yet believed" (John 20:29). Jesus' advice is similar to what we find in Exodus 15:26.

Healing can only come if we obey God's word. And so, Jesus offers us words of eternal life that save us from a horrible damnation. Will we not believe? And will not our belief demand that we trust His words for eternal life? Now is the time to pursue knowing the Lord Your Healer, Jehovah Rophe, through Jesus Christ.

> "My sheep hear My voice, and I know them, and they follow Me; and I give eternal life to them, and they shall never perish; and no one shall snatch them out of My hand" (John 10:27-28).

#13 Study Questions

How should I or others face the possibility of death through sickness?

1. How would you finish the statement? We are all 100% guaranteed to _____?

2. Why is it that all people die?

3. Some cultures believe it is not good to talk about death, but why is it helpful to talk about the possibility of death?

4. Does anyone really want to die? (Even those who choose death would rather have life if it was possible.)

5. Why is the fatalism connected to: "If I get the disease, then I will not fight it" wrong?

6. How does Hezekiah show in Isaiah 38 that it is okay to seek life?

7. Why is faith necessary to genuinely pray and ask God for health?

8. Why should hospitals upfront provide the associated costs for operations and treatments?

9. Is it right to go into serious debt for healing? What is the consequence of this debt?

10. What principles can help guide us while trying to preserve a person's life or to allow him or her to die?

11. What does it mean by stating that we should treat any serious sickness as a time to encounter the Healer? How does it work out? What should we expect?

12. Why is healing only temporary? What does Jesus offer in John 10:27-28? How do these differ?

13. How might I kindly speak to someone going through a difficult medical crisis?

Appendix 1: Audio Summaries

Each question has a special audio summary along with a prayer to strengthen our confidence in our Healer! Scroll down to the end for the continuous soundtrack for traveling (90 minutes). Download this page with the soundtrack links at bit.ly/lyh-audio or scan the QR code below with your smartphone.[13]

---

[13] Contact author via email on page 4 for any problems.

About the Author

Rev. Paul J. Bucknell, an active author and international instructor, has written more than twenty books on pertinent Christian training topics. His books are written with the conviction that the more we build our lives on the truth of God's Word, the stronger and more vibrant our faith and lives will be. Paul's international training seminars take God's Word and apply the truth therein to different aspects of Christian living for pastors and Christian leaders. As founder of Biblical Foundations for Freedom, Paul provides printed and digital media along with video training courses and an ongoing website ministry. Paul with his wife, Linda, are still busy raising eight children and presently delight in having four grandchildren.

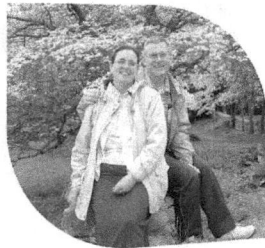

(More on Paul, Linda, and the ministry)[14]

---

[14] http://www.foundationsforfreedom.net/Help/AboutBFF/Biography.html